THE STORM
IS IN THE MIND
NOT IN YOU

Title: The Storm Is In The Mind, Not In You
ISBN: 9798993919584

- *Some places in the book use "Ex." as an abbreviation for the word "Example."*
- *The character 'Bean' featured throughout this book is a fictional composite created by the author solely for illustrative and educational purposes.*

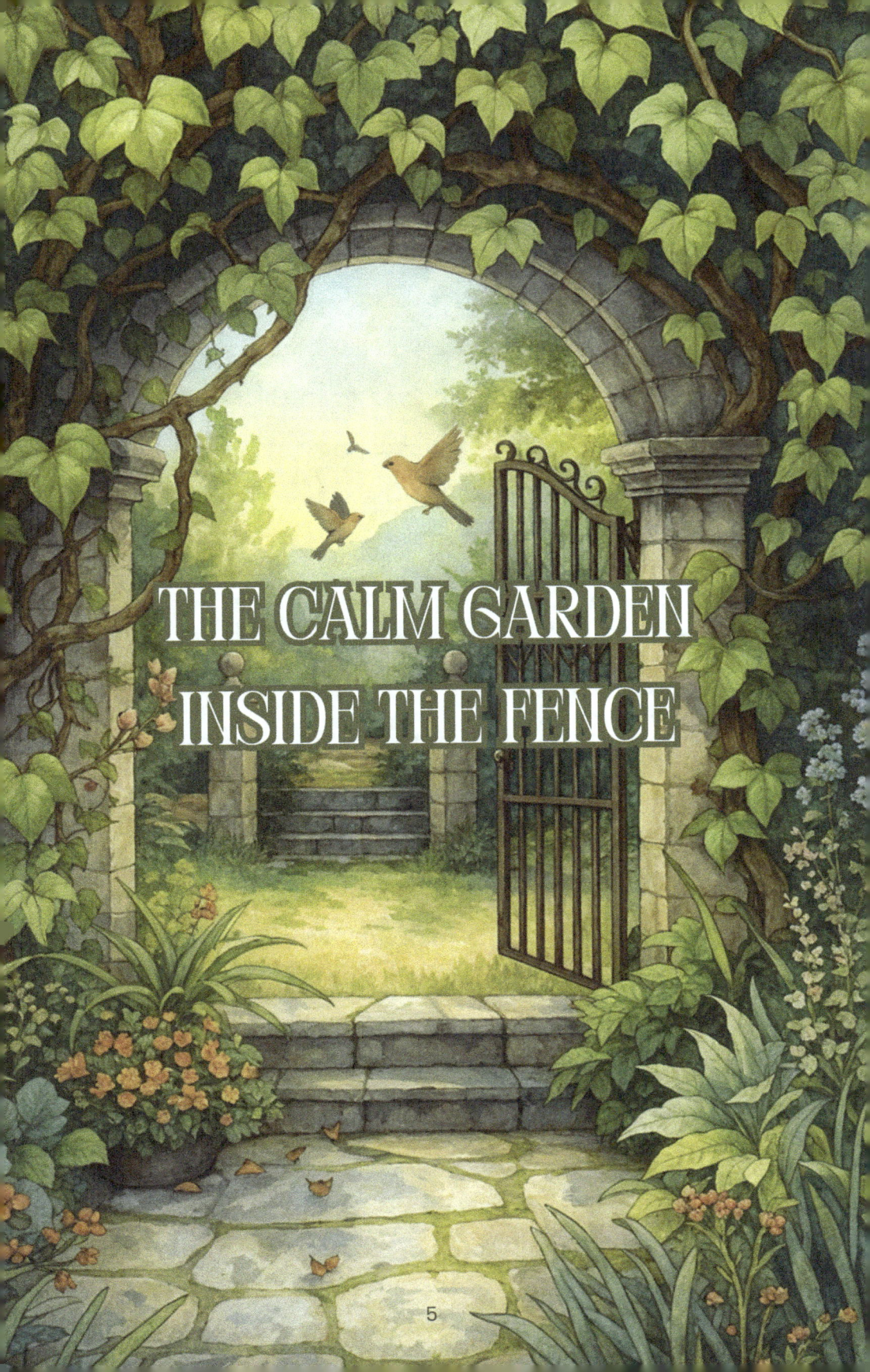

THE CALM GARDEN
INSIDE THE FENCE

Imagine that you are stepping into a beautiful garden. The garden is surrounded by a tall, strong, and steady fence. Once you close the gate, imagine all noise and negativity staying outside, whether they come from voices, people, or events that have happened or are still happening in your life. The gate and the fence are your guardians.

Inside the garden, the atmosphere is quiet and peaceful. Warm sunlight gently touches your skin. Imagine worries beginning to soften and fade here. You decide what belongs in this garden. It may be your heart, your soul, your mind. Around you are trees, grass, flowers, and leaves filled with living color, waiting for your care so they can grow more vibrant each day. You walk closer and touch the plants and flowers, feeling your connection to the goodness you may have once overlooked. No one else tends this garden. You are the one who nourishes it.

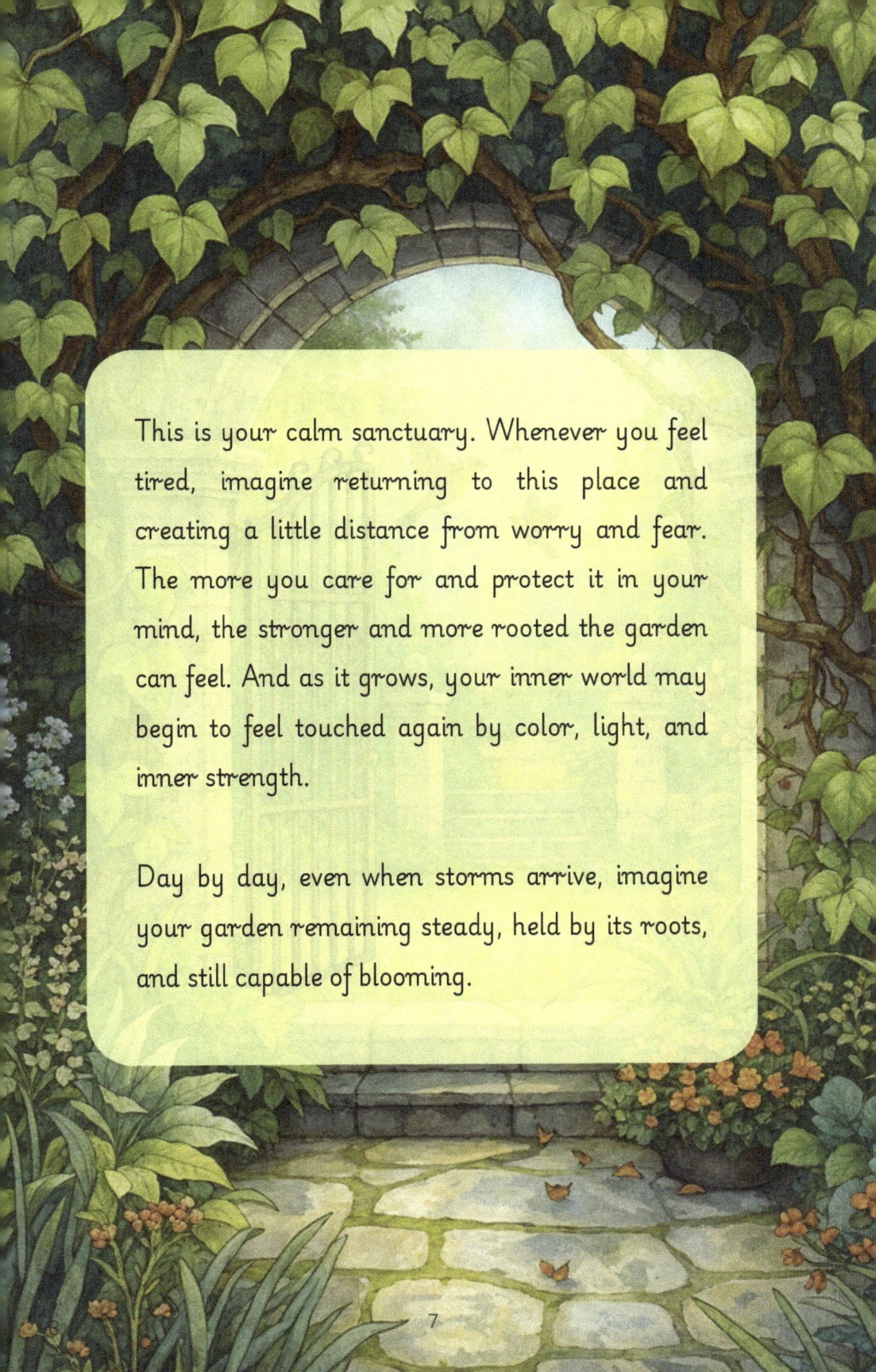

This is your calm sanctuary. Whenever you feel tired, imagine returning to this place and creating a little distance from worry and fear. The more you care for and protect it in your mind, the stronger and more rooted the garden can feel. And as it grows, your inner world may begin to feel touched again by color, light, and inner strength.

Day by day, even when storms arrive, imagine your garden remaining steady, held by its roots, and still capable of blooming.

CHAPTER 1

THE STORM THAT NEVER STOPS
SPINNING IN THE MIND

There are times when we are inside an inner storm without even realizing it. We only feel endlessly tired and heavy inside, until our energy slowly runs out without us even knowing when it happened. The busyness and pressure of life leave us without even a single moment to pause and bring ourselves into a state still enough to see that a storm is spinning in the mind. There are also times when we know we are living inside that storm, but we do not know where to begin. And so we simply let the storm control our life by default.

But when we see the storm as a flow of movement with traces, with a starting point, a continuation point, and a result, it becomes less vague and clearer. Instead of letting the storm silently lead our emotions, we learn to stop, observe, and recognize each small spiral inside it that makes it spin.

For example, there is a person named Bean who often has the thought, "I'm too tired. There is no way I can get through this." After that, Bean avoids pursuing the things he once felt passionate about. As a result, Bean feels disappointed and powerless about his life.

Spiral 1 - What I thought -> Spiral 2 - What I did -> Spiral 3 - What happened

At this point, what appears after Spiral 3 in Bean's example? Usually, after the "What happened," the mind returns to a new line of thought or repeats the original line of thought. In this way, the storm keeps spinning again and again in its own cycle.

When we observe the inner storm as a structure made of small spirals, we begin to feel less unclear. Perhaps it is no longer as frightening, too enormous, or everlasting as we once thought. Instead of being swept away by the storm, we begin to see a possibility, however small, that brings something different: even if it is only the act of seeing it, the whole storm may no longer spin in the same old way.

For example, instead of letting a negative thought push Bean to give up on a passion, he can acknowledge his line of thought and still return to that passion, even without motivation. This small shift in the storm's spiral may somehow open space for possibility, the possibility of change, instead of assuming that he is permanently trapped in the spiral.

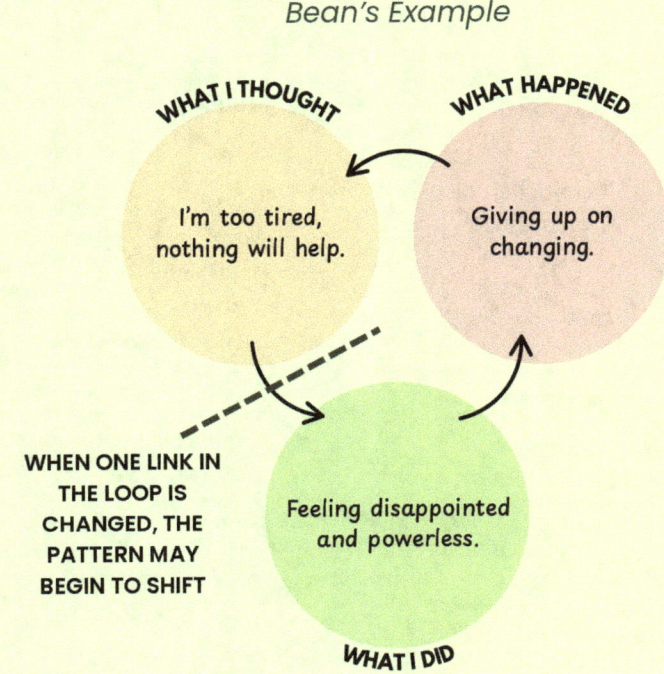

Bean's Example

WHAT I THOUGHT

I'm too tired, nothing will help.

WHAT HAPPENED

Giving up on changing.

WHEN ONE LINK IN THE LOOP IS CHANGED, THE PATTERN MAY BEGIN TO SHIFT

Feeling disappointed and powerless.

WHAT I DID

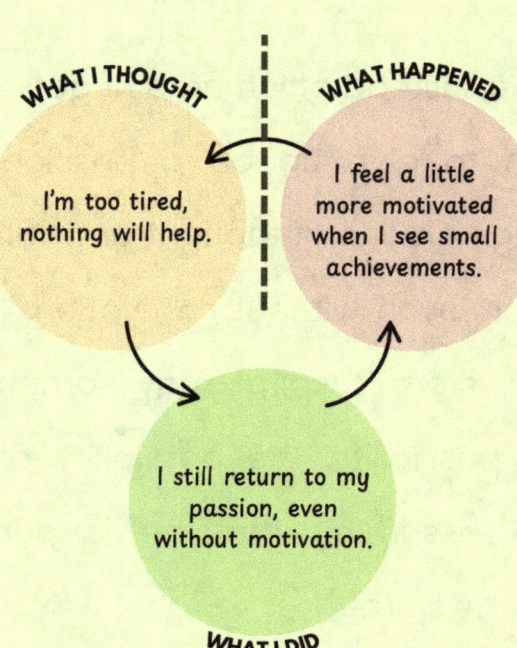

WHAT I THOUGHT

I'm too tired, nothing will help.

WHAT HAPPENED

I feel a little more motivated when I see small achievements.

I still return to my passion, even without motivation.

WHAT I DID

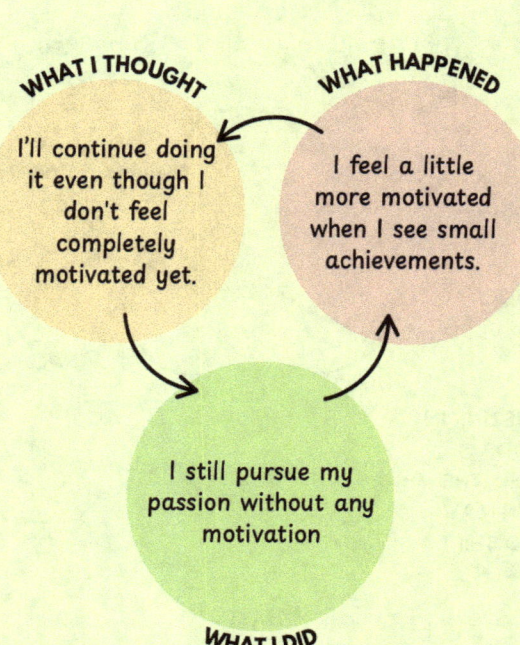

WHAT I THOUGHT

I'll continue doing it even though I don't feel completely motivated yet.

WHAT HAPPENED

I feel a little more motivated when I see small achievements.

I still pursue my passion without any motivation

WHAT I DID

CHAPTER 2

THE DEEPER STORIES HIDDEN BENEATH EACH LINE OF THOUGHT

"It's my fault."

"I'll never get through this."

"Everything is against me."

We often drown in wandering thoughts that repeat over and over, day after day, but have we ever asked ourselves whether there is a story hidden beneath that line of thought? If we stop and ask ourselves what led us to that thought, we seem to begin to realize that there is a deep belief leading to that line of thought, and behind that belief, there exists another layer called "fear." When we find the fear, we can name it and observe it for a long time in order to understand ourselves more deeply.

Beliefs and fears lie hidden beneath many layers of emotion. Because we have never searched for them or named them, we keep drowning in the top layer of "wandering thoughts." We did not even choose them, yet they may still exist somewhere deep inside our hearts without needing anyone's permission. But sadly, beliefs and fears seem to be able to shape the way we see the world around us.

"I'm useless."

"I'm not worthy."

"I'm not good enough to keep what is good."

For example, when we think that if we live honestly with our own emotions, the people around us will leave. This belief can make us always live with caution and hesitation in everyday life. We begin to worry about being left by the people we trust, and sometimes we may even have to wear a mask to live, until we grow further and further away from our true self. But what is not real usually does not last long, and then it makes us struggle and suffer in our mind. If we keep letting beliefs and fears exist, then day after day, month after month, we gradually believe in them as a truth without ever asking whether they are still suitable for who we are in the present.

But there is one interesting thing: when we begin to carry an old belief, it may be because we once tried to protect ourselves from a wound in the past. For example, in the past, when we were in a difficult situation and were once abandoned, we began to believe that everyone would leave us. But as time passes, that difficult situation may no longer be the same as before, and we may have become stronger, more resilient in our soul. Yet the belief that "everyone will eventually abandon me" still continues to exist somewhere in the heart, limiting us, causing us to keep circling around fear.

A belief is like a covering that wraps around us and keeps us in one place, not letting us step outside. But now, when we begin to find the deep fear beneath it, we can gradually peel that covering away, little by little.

For example, when we ask:

If that belief were truly right, what fear would it reveal?

Line of thought <- Belief <- Fear

Line of thought <- Belief <- Fear

For example, Bean often has the thought that he will ruin the meeting (Line of thought), because he always believes that he is a failure (Belief), and this belief may be connected to a memory from school, when he was criticized each time he made mistakes many times (Fear).

LINE OF THOUGHT	FEAR
I'm a failure.	I often made mistakes in the past.

Bean's Example

From Bean's example, we learn that a belief can be learned when we try to adapt or fit into a certain environment. It is not necessarily our nature, and it is not necessarily something eternal. Understanding this, we can try to learn a new belief that is more balanced, like taking off old clothes that we once wore in winter to protect ourselves from the cold. Now that summer has come, we need cooler clothes that are more suitable for the version of ourselves in the present.

Now, when Bean understands this, he will learn a new belief by reading aloud every day:

This is a belief I learned. It may not reflect the full truth.

As Bean relearns the new belief until it gradually softens the old belief, he begins the first steps of wearing new clothes, and realizes that wearing winter clothes in summer is not a command. It is a choice.

Bean's Example

HIDDEN BELIEF   >>>   **REMINDER**

I'm a failure.

This is a belief I learned. It may not reflect the full truth.

HIDDEN BELIEF   >>>   **REMINDER**

I'll never get through this.

This is a belief I learned. It may not reflect the full truth.

CHAPTER 3

WHEN WE MISTAKE THE STORM FOR THE WHOLE TRUTH

Have there ever been times when, inside an inner storm, we asked ourselves whether we and the storm are two separate things, rather than one and the same?

Returning to Bean's example, when he begins to question whether the storm may not be the whole truth, Bean slowly sees that he is no longer one with the storm. Instead, a small distance between Bean and the storm begins to appear. Bean no longer stands in the center of the storm and becomes one with it, as if he belongs to the storm. Instead, Bean begins to stand in a different place outside the storm.

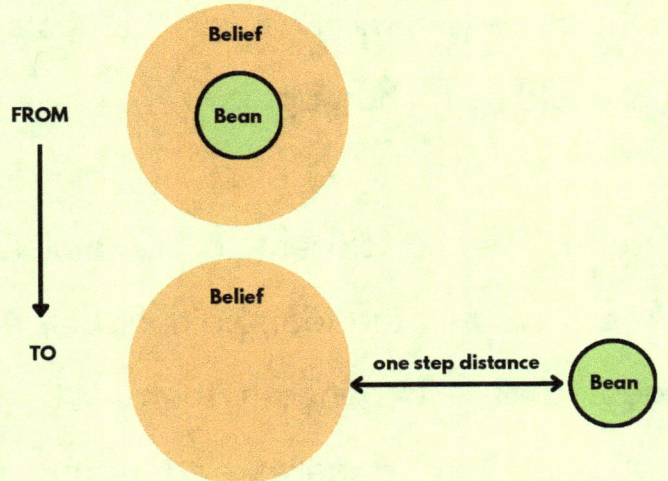

Bean's Example

Here, Bean sees a new perspective: The storm is not the whole of who he is. It is not his identity. The storm is not his deepest self. It is more like fences formed around old fears during times when he was trying to protect himself and move through what felt painful, uncertain, or difficult. The storm is not always the enemy. In many cases, it reflects earlier efforts to avoid being hurt again.

When Bean listened closely to his beliefs, they sometimes revealed the fear, pain, or unmet need that seemed to live beneath them. When Bean stepped back from a belief and returned to a steadier sense of self beyond it, the belief began to feel less dominant in the way he saw himself.

From "I'm inside the belief."
→ To "I'm the observer watching the belief, not the one fully merged with it."

Are we truly that storm? Or can we still choose to step into another position, far enough to observe it? And when our point of view begins to change, the storm seems to no longer bind us completely as it once did.

That is why, when we change the position from which we observe a problem, we often discover new things about our own inner world.

When we are inside a heavy line of thought, there are times when we feel as if we have become one with it. Something inside us remains trapped in some dark corner, as if that is the default, as if that is the whole truth. But when we begin to ask ourselves whether we are attaching ourselves to the center of the storm, a small distance begins to appear. Are we truly that storm? Or can we still choose to step into another position, far enough to observe it? And when our point of view begins to change, the storm seems to no longer bind us completely as it once did. That is why, when we change the position from which we observe a problem, we often discover new things about our own inner world.

What is this new thing? Let us return to Bean's story. After he leaves his old position and steps outside to observe the storm, he begins to "ask" the storm:

"Hey, are you truly the whole truth?"

Then Bean begins to ask himself:

"What makes me believe that this storm is the whole truth?"

"Am I exaggerating this storm too much?"

"If so, what might reveal another side of this storm that I have overlooked?"

Next, he answers these three questions himself.

For example, Bean has a belief that:

I will never succeed because others always criticize me.

"What makes me believe that this storm is the whole truth?"

→ I have received harsh comments from coworkers and family about my choices.

"Am I exaggerating this storm too much?"

→ It seems so.

"If so, what might reveal another side of this storm that I have overlooked?"

→ I have also received positive feedback. Some criticism was about specific situations, not my whole ability. Constructive comments can help me grow.

After answering the third question, Bean is startled because he has discovered something he seems to have forgotten. It is not necessarily that it does not exist. It is just that the things proving the belief that he will always be criticized have become too dominant, so they have overwhelmed the things proving the opposite. And then the old belief he has always held keeps repeating like a film, until it becomes so convincing that it feels almost like the whole truth.

Returning again to Bean's story, he continues to relearn a more balanced belief based on the old belief.

For example:
Bean's old belief: "I always fail."
A more balanced way to see it: "Sometimes I fail, but I also succeed. One failure does not erase the moments when I did well."

Although the storm gradually calms down, he is still not truly used to the new belief. But that is okay. Something new often needs time to become familiar, like planting a new seed and letting time help it sprout.

Example

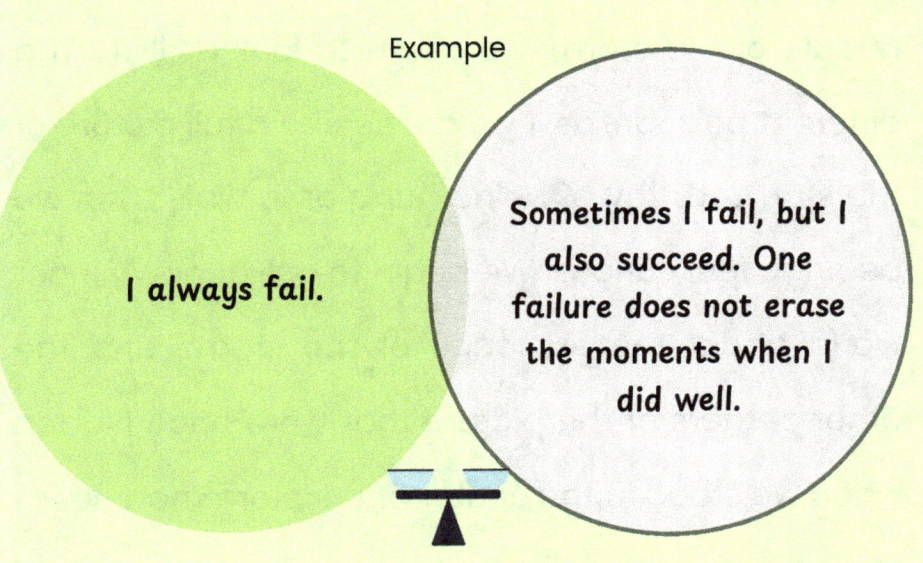

I always fail.

Sometimes I fail, but I also succeed. One failure does not erase the moments when I did well.

When we no longer see ourselves as being in the middle of the storm, we begin to look at it from a different position, as if we are seeing a full picture of the storm worthy of being hung on a wall. Then we begin to feel curious. We begin to ask our own inner world about the existence of the storm, and the other corners of the picture that were once hidden when we stood in the center of the storm now seem to become a little clearer as we look at the picture from a distance.

CHAPTER 4

BETWEEN WHAT WE SEE AND WHAT WE FEEL

The storm in the mind can sometimes act like clouded mirrors, changing the way we see a situation. For example, we may fail once at something and then begin to expect the future to fail as well. A simple event, which may have started as only one part of a much larger picture, can slowly become stretched, narrowed, or reshaped inside us until it no longer feels connected to the larger picture.

This may happen because the present moment sometimes carries traces of earlier experiences, especially if criticism, disappointment, or hurt have been repeated many times in the past. But the past is not the whole of who we are. The version of us that once stood in those moments has continued to change over time. We learn, we adapt, and we do not always return to life in exactly the same way.

Sometimes, the storm inside us can feel as if there is a prophet within us, turning intuition into worry, and worry into a trap. For example, we may predict that today will be just as difficult as yesterday because the days before have already felt heavy. This may leave little room for change or surprise.

But one thing remains true: no one can predict the future with complete certainty. No matter how convincing a fear may sound, there are always variables we cannot fully see. So whenever the storm begins predicting something terrible, it may help to remember that uncertainty also leaves room for another possibility.

The storm inside us can also treat one painful moment in life as if it were enough to define the entire future. Life holds both light and darkness. That is what makes it life. Darkness helps us recognize light. If we were born and only ever saw light, how would we know the difference between good and bad? For example, if we never failed, how would we notice that a method we once followed was not right for us, and that another path might fit better?

Not everything painful has to be treated as meaningless. Some experiences become part of how we learn, adjust, and keep growing over time.

The storm inside us can also appear when we start assuming what other people are thinking or feeling without truly knowing.

Once again, remember this:

We cannot know everything just by following habit, fear, or old pain from the past. And even if we could somehow read other people's thoughts, their thoughts still would not be a final or reliable definition of who we are.

In many cases, when we start guessing what others are thinking, it can also reveal something about the way we see ourselves. And if that self-image has been shaped by a heavy thought, we can return to Bean's example, where he asked:

"Hey, are you truly the whole truth?"

Then Bean begins to ask himself:

"What makes me believe that this storm is the whole truth?"

"Am I exaggerating this storm too much?"

"If so, what might reveal another side of this storm that I have overlooked?"

When we understand these kinds of inner storms, we may realize that a thought can sound convincing inside us and still fail to reflect the full picture. Over time, we may become more able to notice when a thought is being shaped by an old storm rather than by the larger picture of the moment. And we may begin creating more space between what we feel and what is true. In this space, there is often more room to choose a response, rather than letting the storm quietly decide for us.

CHAPTER 5

DESIGN A CALM GARDEN

Imagine that you are stepping into a beautiful garden. The garden is surrounded by a tall, strong, and steady fence. Once you close the gate, imagine all noise and negativity staying outside, whether they come from voices, people, or events that have happened or are still happening in your life. The gate and the fence are your guardians.

Inside the garden, the atmosphere is quiet and peaceful. Warm sunlight gently touches your skin. Imagine worries beginning to soften and fade here. You decide what belongs in this garden. It may be your heart, your soul, your mind. Around you are trees, grass, flowers, and leaves filled with living color, waiting for your care so they can grow more vibrant each day. You walk closer and touch the plants and flowers, feeling your connection to the goodness you may have once overlooked. No one else tends this garden. You are the one who nourishes it.

This is your calm sanctuary. Whenever you feel tired, imagine returning to this place and creating a little distance from worry and fear. The more you care for and protect it in your mind, the stronger and more rooted the garden can feel. And as it grows, your inner world may begin to feel touched again by color, light, and inner strength.

Each time you return to your garden, through your care and tending, the trees grow greener and stronger. Their roots can become a gentle reminder of the resilience you are trying to nurture within yourself. Day by day, even when storms arrive, imagine your garden remaining steady, held by its roots, and still capable of blooming.

Start by imagining the overall feeling of your garden: Is it wide and open like a soft meadow that makes you feel free? Or is it small and intimate like a warm tea garden that gives you a sense of protection?

Is your garden bright and lively like the light of early morning? Or shaded and cool like a quiet path through a deep green forest?

Move closer to the gate and the fence: What are they made of that makes them feel strong and secure? How tall would you like them to be so they feel protective to you? Could they even cover the sky, if that would help you feel more sheltered during a storm? Is the fence the color of warm wood, or pure white?

Now step inside and look at the objects within your garden:

- A tall ancient tree with roots deep in the earth may represent your steady inner core, your discipline, and your strength that is not easily shaken by outside pressure.
- A still pond may represent the calm and quiet you find in your breath.
- A chair resting under the sunlight may represent rest and the gentle warmth that soothes your heart.

PLAN FOR MY DESIGN

What color is it?
Ex. Soft golden light, like sunrise after rain.

What sounds do you hear there?
Ex. Wind through tall trees, a stream whispering nearby.

What protects the space around you?
Ex. A wall of vines and sunlight that filters the noise.

What does it protect you from?
Ex. Old fears, harsh voices, and rushing thoughts.

Who or what do you allow to enter?
Ex. My breath, quiet moments, the warmth of calm.

What do you plant or grow there?
Ex. Seeds of trust that grow a little more each time I visit.

CHAPTER 6

FIND PEACE IN MOMENTS OF CHAOS AND UNCERTAINTY

When we are inside emotional chaos, we seem to want to find some kind of clarity to drive away the blurry fog, ultimately so we can find a sense of reassurance about something. Sometimes we even become so burdened by painful experiences from the past that even a one percent chance of danger feels unacceptable. In moments like that, what the mind often seems to be seeking is relief, and certainty can create the feeling of relief. Certainty may bring us a sense of calm because it creates the illusion of control.

What often keeps worry alive may not be uncertainty itself, but the constant struggle to get rid of it. We may keep reaching for certainty because we want to make everything predictable. When that does not happen, uncertainty can start to feel like something is wrong, and that feeling may pull us further into worry and control.

A sense of relief may begin when we stop using certainty as our only form of protection. This does not mean that we should welcome risky situations or ignore real warning signs. The point here is something else: to let uncertainty exist without automatically seeing it as something that will only lead to suffering. It is like a closed book. We cannot read every page all at once, but the book is not dangerous simply because it is closed. It may hold other possibilities too.

Up to this point, we have begun looking at uncertainty from a different angle. Now we begin to explore how to shift our relationship with uncertainty. Instead of seeing it only as an enemy that brings worry, something that must always be overcome, we can begin to see it as a companion that may also carry curiosity and unexpected possibilities.

When we stop demanding certain answers about the future, we create a small space where hope, flexibility, and growth can exist. Before, when we looked at uncertainty, it may have seemed as if only risk was there. Now, possibility is there too.

Imagine a dark room filled only with fear about the mistakes that might happen. Now imagine another quiet voice entering that room, a voice that carries a different kind of openness. For example, when we are learning to ride a bicycle, instead of believing that the only possible outcome is falling, we begin to allow another possibility: that we might ride even one turn of the wheel without falling.

Life may never come with one hundred percent certainty, and yet we have already made our way through countless unknowns. Even while carrying fear, we have still made it to today. We have still learned, changed, and discovered many things along the way. And when we begin to see uncertainty as part of life, rather than a problem we must exhaust ourselves trying to predict, it may begin to feel a little less overwhelming than it once did.

Bean's Example

ORIGINAL:

"What if the next day
goes badly?"

REFRAME:

"I can't know for sure, and
that means it could also
go smoothly, or better
than I expect."

CHAPTER 7

BEFRIEND THE STORM WITHIN

There may be a voice of the storm within us, and it often says things like: "You will never be good enough."

Sometimes this voice keeps repeating in our mind. Little by little, it becomes so familiar that it starts to feel convincing. We follow it and believe it without even realizing when it happened. But when we fight against it, we may only grow more tense or try to run away from it. On the other hand, when we try to sit down, listen, and gently befriend the storm within, we may begin to understand why it appears.

We can understand what fear led to the voice of the storm. Sometimes this voice exists because it wants to remind us of our mistakes in the past, so we can avoid making the same mistakes again. But over time, it may also make it hard to touch peace, because we keep living in the fear of making mistakes.

After that, we learn how to befriend the voice of the storm in the mind.

Befriending the storm? It may not sound very useful, but in truth, it can create a wider space in the mind. Instead of having only one crowded room bound by a voice that belongs to the past, we now have a little more space for what has been renewed over time. Instead of being bound by fear, shame, and failure, now a more balanced voice appears, opening up space for learning and growth.

Bean's Example:

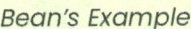

I'm going nowhere.

I'm moving slower than I expected, not standing still. Progress doesn't always look like growth. Sometimes it looks like staying alive and not giving up.

Imagine that a friend, or even a stranger, came to us and told us about their mistakes and failures from the past. How would we respond? I guess most of us are not harsh enough to blame someone who is already hurting. More often, we try to comfort them, empathize with them, and encourage them with words that feel warm and strengthening. We choose our language carefully so they will feel less wounded.

But the strange irony is that we often do not do the same for ourselves. We might say to someone else, "Try not to keep living in the past. You have already been so strong." And yet, when something similar happens to us, the voice of the storm within us may become heavy, saying things like, "I'm a failure," or "I should never do this again." The tone changes as if we have turned against ourselves, severe and impatient.

By learning to treat ourselves the way we would treat someone we love, we may begin to step back from this trap of harsh self-judgment that can quietly form inside us. If the voice of the storm notices only the mistakes and forgets the strengths, the friend's voice remembers both. It sees the mistakes and the strengths, and it also makes room for guidance and care.

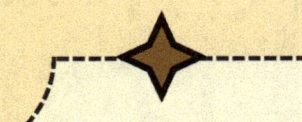

Dear present me,

I know you are still carrying burdens from the past, and even now, they still echo inside you. But no matter what, you still have the right to keep living today. None of us were born to become a perfect version of ourselves from the very beginning. And yet, from those imperfect pieces, the person you are now was formed, more mature and stronger inside. Painful stories are proof that you have survived well up to this moment. They do not define your whole identity.

Remember never to label yourself with any fixed measure of worth. You are simply you, just as the stars in the universe never ask where they belong, and the ocean never asks how wide it is. Nothing creates a definition of your worth, and nothing can, except the labels you place on yourself.

Whenever negative thoughts appear again, remember the times you were strong enough to make it through the storms in your life.

With steady care,
Your wiser self

Example

MY SOOTHING PHRASES

Write short sentences you can repeat to yourself when low:

CHAPTER 8

THE STORM OF SELF-BLAME

When life feels frightening, unstable, or hard to understand, something inside us may respond in ways that seem protective. Sometimes self-blame becomes one of those responses. It can create a sense of control, as if naming ourselves as the cause might make fear feel smaller, clearer, or easier to contain. In moments like that, it can begin to seem as though the problem is us.

An unanswered message. Our feelings were dismissed. A series of painful moments arriving all at once, almost like punishment. Or one contemptuous remark that continues to echo inside us. Little by little, these moments can gather into a single conclusion: It is my fault. Sometimes that conclusion may reflect an earlier way of trying to make sense of pain.

If life came in only two colors, light and darkness, then light might hold the achievement, while darkness might hold pain, failure, and the shame that can grow around them. But none of us lives a life made only of light. All the colors of life help shape who we are becoming, carrying both pain and wisdom within them.

We should not expect some kind of magic that removes shame all at once. Here, softening shame means changing the way we respond to it. When a shame-filled voice appears, we do not have to believe it immediately. The moment we stop accepting it as truth right away, we create a little more space to pause, to understand, and to trace where it may be coming from. Beneath the pain, we may begin to notice something that has been there for a long time: old places inside us that were never fully seen or understood.

Why do we so often blame ourselves? Sometimes it becomes a way of staying alert, of trying to predict pain before it arrives. Understanding why shame takes root, and why it stays, may help us see that much of it may grow from hidden beliefs shaped by difficult experiences rather than from the full truth of who we are. Even that realization may begin to loosen shame.

When we do not separate the voice of shame from reality, it may grow so certain of itself that it sounds like a truth carved in stone. The voice of shame often acts as if judging us first might protect us from being hurt again. It may still believe that if it criticizes us first, we will be less shaken when others seem ready to do the same.

Meet it as we would meet a frightened child, with calm eyes and open hands ready to offer warmth. Remember this short sentence, if you can, so we can say it back to our inner alarm whenever it rises:

"I know you are trying to help in your own way, but I do not need that kind of protection now."

Our old stories may have cost us many good things, dreams we had not yet had the chance to pursue, and opportunities we might have used to rebuild our life. Once we see that more clearly, we can begin writing a new story about shame. Let it remind us that the old story does not define the value of our life in the present, and it is not the same as who we are now. The old story can also remind us that we endured, that we made it through those moments to arrive here, and that we are still moving toward a future with greater inner strength.

Just a small reminder:

You do not need to become valuable to deserve anything. Human beings created the label of value through social standards that people use to judge one another. The sky does not measure itself. The stars do not compete for their place. Everything that comes into being exists simply as itself.

If you feel tired of always having to prove who you are, or of trying to become good enough to exist without guilt, let this be a reminder that you are allowed to lay that burden down. You were never born to justify your existence.

CHAPTER 9

THE "ME" THAT WAS ALREADY ENOUGH

Perfectionism can become one of the forces that keeps the inner storm spinning. Many people find themselves caught in loops like these:

Feeling "not enough" → fear and hesitation → procrastination and waiting → not seeing the results they hoped for, not feeling any real sense of reward → feeling heavier inside → feeling even more lost in the storm.

Feeling "not enough" → putting excessive pressure on themselves, racing against time → exhaustion → not seeing the results they hoped for, not feeling any real sense of reward → feeling heavier inside → struggling even more with the storm within.

What brings you happiness from the deepest part of your soul is your true measure of success, not something that exists only to be recognized by others or something you have to strain yourself to prove. For some people, simply becoming a person with a pure heart who does not harm anyone is already success, because they feel peace in their spirit each day instead of resentment or anger.

Do not define success only as becoming someone valuable by someone else's standards, such as being rich, having high status in society, or maintaining an image of worth in a relationship. It may be worth pausing before believing everything social media repeats about the so-called "value of a man" or the "value of a woman."

If you begin to strip away the labels of value that you have been carrying every day, you may gradually feel a little more space inside.

What is it that makes you happy from deep within? Pause for a moment to reflect, and write it here. Remember it whenever you feel lost or overwhelmed in this busy world.

.....60s.....

Learning to accept what is "good enough" may help us step out of the old spiral little by little. Perfectionism begins to become a problem when it keeps feeding the inner storm. At that point, it is often connected to fear of judgment, fear of failure, fear of being left behind, in short, fear.

When we begin to believe that only a perfect outcome can give us **peace**, nothing seems allowed to exist except perfection. We may become unable to rest, as if one mistake could ruin everything. The pursuit of perfection can sometimes come from a desire to feel safe, but it can also bring heaviness with it.

Accepting what is "good enough" means:
Gradually loosening the belief that our peace or worth depends on perfection.

Often, perfectionism is not only about striving for excellence. It can also come from the fear that everything will collapse if something goes wrong. It can make a person feel as though one mistake could ruin everything, so waiting, or doing nothing at all, may seem like the only way to avoid making things worse.

Now, we begin to practice acting without waiting for perfection, while slowly opening ourselves to a different way of seeing things: taking action does not always mean something will go wrong, and imperfection does not determine our worth.

Put simply, perhaps worth is not something that exists to measure a human being in the first place. You are simply you, just as a star in the sky does not fight for its place in the universe. It simply is.

THE PERFECTION MONSTER

Bean's Example

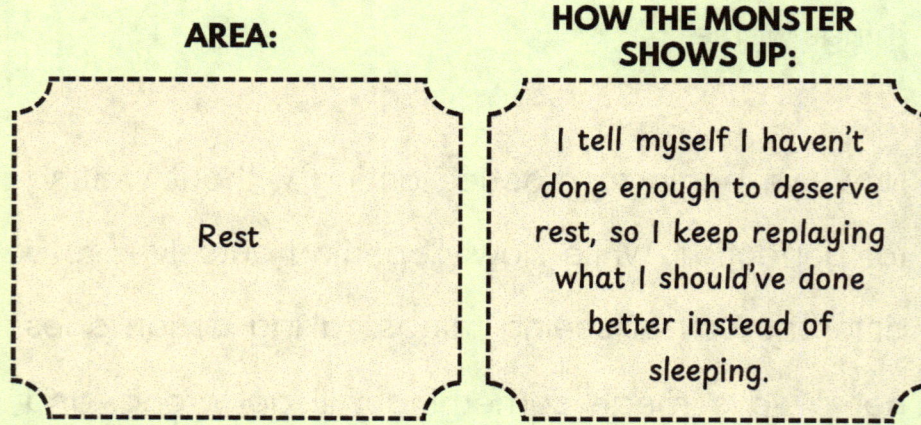

AREA:

Rest

HOW THE MONSTER SHOWS UP:

I tell myself I haven't done enough to deserve rest, so I keep replaying what I should've done better instead of sleeping.

IMPACT ON ME:

My mind keeps looping, I can't truly rest.

Redefine Success

Instead of seeing success as something far too high to reach, try lowering that standard to a place that feels more comfortable to you. For example, instead of telling yourself that you must make one billion dollars before you can call yourself rich, try thinking more simply: being able to breathe, stand here, and continue today is already a form of success.

When we look at perfectionistic thoughts from a softer place, we open ourselves to a different way of seeing life, instead of letting the inner struggle around perfection run on by itself. As that struggle becomes clearer, we may start to see what has been shaping it. The harsh rules we once lived by may gradually give way to standards that feel more balanced and easier to live with.

Over time, our definition of success may shift from chasing perfect outcomes to valuing the process of living, with all its surprises, rises, and falls, and most importantly, to living more honestly with what truly brings us happiness deep within.

PERFECTIONISTIC THOUGHT

BALANCED STANDARD

I must never make mistakes in presentations.

What matters is sharing my ideas clearly.

I tell myself I haven't done enough to deserve rest, so I keep replaying what I should've done better instead of sleeping.

I'm allowed to rest even when things are unfinished.

CHAPTER 10

INNER STRENGTH

Imagine we listen to a different kind of voice that has also been living within us, but may have been forgotten during the time we were hurting. If the first voice is the critic that sees only our mistakes and failures, then the second voice is the encourager, the one that has been witnessing our effort, resilience, and growth through those mistakes, all the way to this present moment.

In the midst of pain, we may feel as though we are falling apart, especially when we lose sight of the difference between pain itself and the evidence that we have endured and made it through. This may happen when the critical voice grows so loud that it drowns out our inner strength. Now is the time to give the second voice space to speak, so that inner strength has a little more room to be heard.

"Even in pain, you're still standing here."

Inner strength is often misunderstood as the ability to stay positive or push through pain without breaking. In reality, inner strength may grow much earlier than that, as it forms in small, quiet moments when we stay with difficult feelings instead of turning against ourselves.

These moments do not feel triumphant, they simply carry the message:
"I can handle this, even if it is hard."

You may begin by sitting with a few memories of the times you made it through something difficult. Do not look only for major achievements. Your strength may be found in something as simple as getting up and trying to begin one more time, even after crying until your eyes were swollen the night before. Or even when you felt exhausted inside, you still made room for kindness by rescuing an abandoned kitten and giving it a chance to live.

Do you notice that you often hear only the criticism, while forgetting memories like these? You may choose three or more inner strengths, signs that even in your exhaustion, you remained strong enough to keep going.

When these words are placed on paper and read again in the future, you may gradually begin to see yourself with a little more fairness.

The more we read them again and again, the more opportunities we create to hear the second voice, the quiet encourager within us, so that the critical voice no longer takes up all the inner space the way it once did.

STRENGTH

I notice when my mind is being harsh, and I pause instead of believing it immediately.

MY STRENGTHS SNAPSHOT

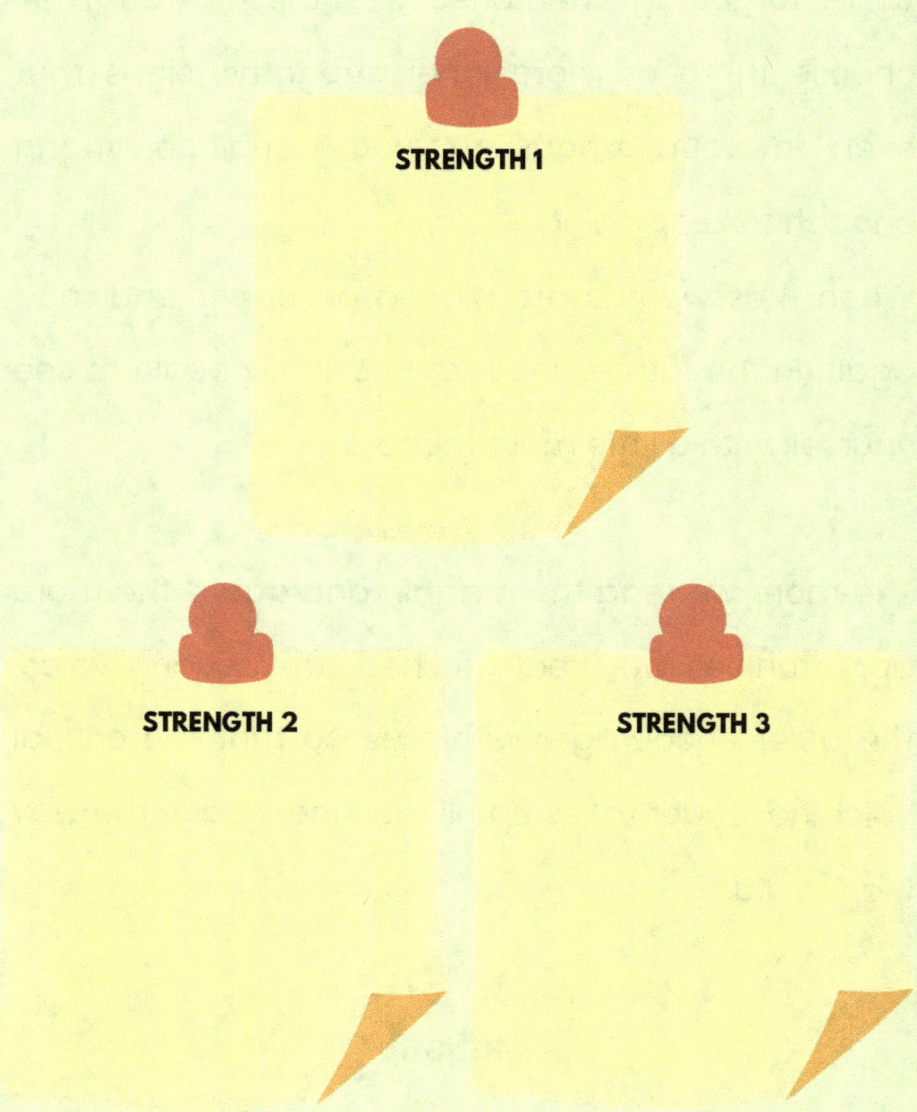

STRENGTH 1

STRENGTH 2

STRENGTH 3

Example:
- Strength 1: I can sit with uncomfortable feelings instead of running away.
- Strength 2: I keep going, even on days when I feel emotionally drained.
- Strength 3: I notice when my mind is being harsh, and I pause instead of believing it immediately.

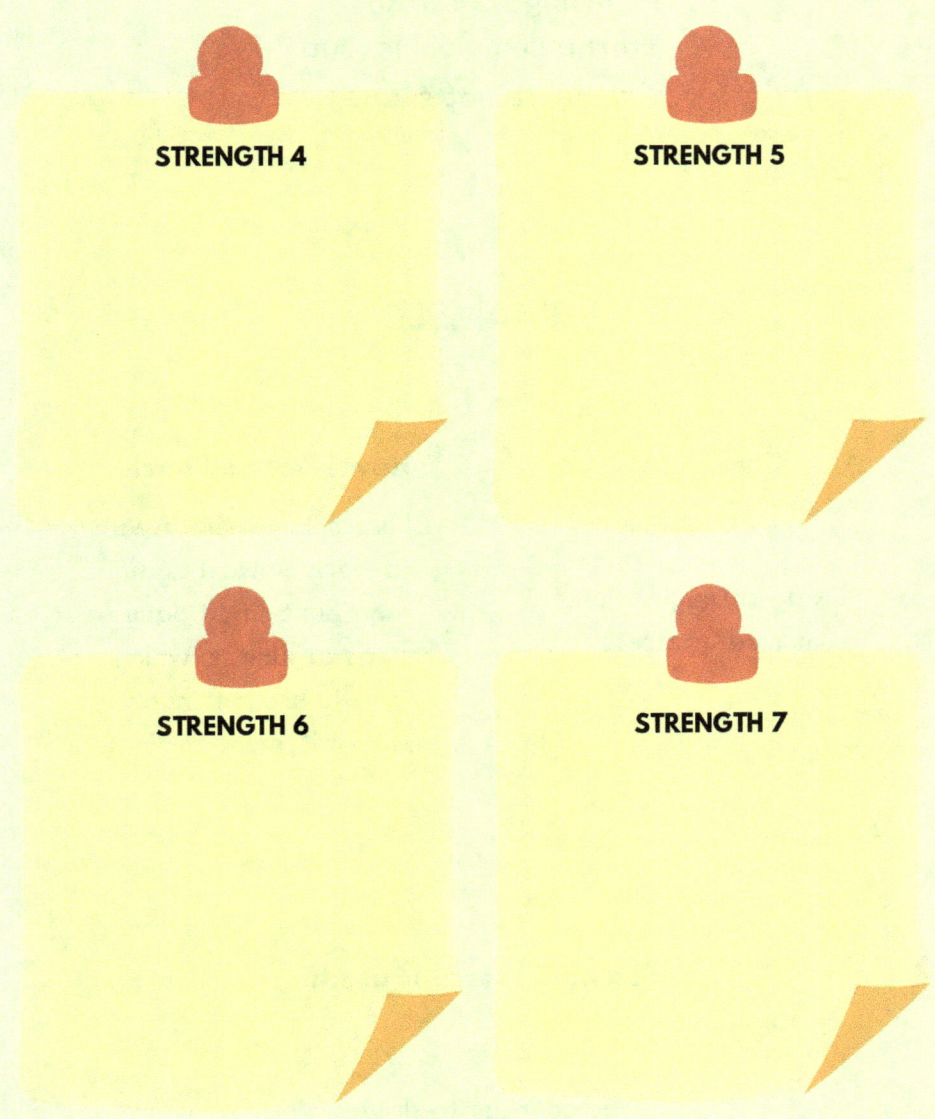

STRENGTH 4

STRENGTH 5

STRENGTH 6

STRENGTH 7

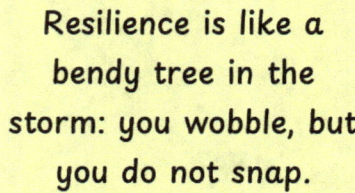

Resilience is like a
bendy tree in the
storm: you wobble, but
you do not snap.

EXAMPLE

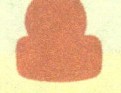

Challenge:

Living through a long
period of stress.

How I crawled back:

Chose a long-held dream
to work toward again
and built small daily
steps around it, which
slowly brought back
excitement for
life

Strength I secretly used:

The courage to dream
again and the steady will
to turn that dream into
action

MY PAST RESILIENCE

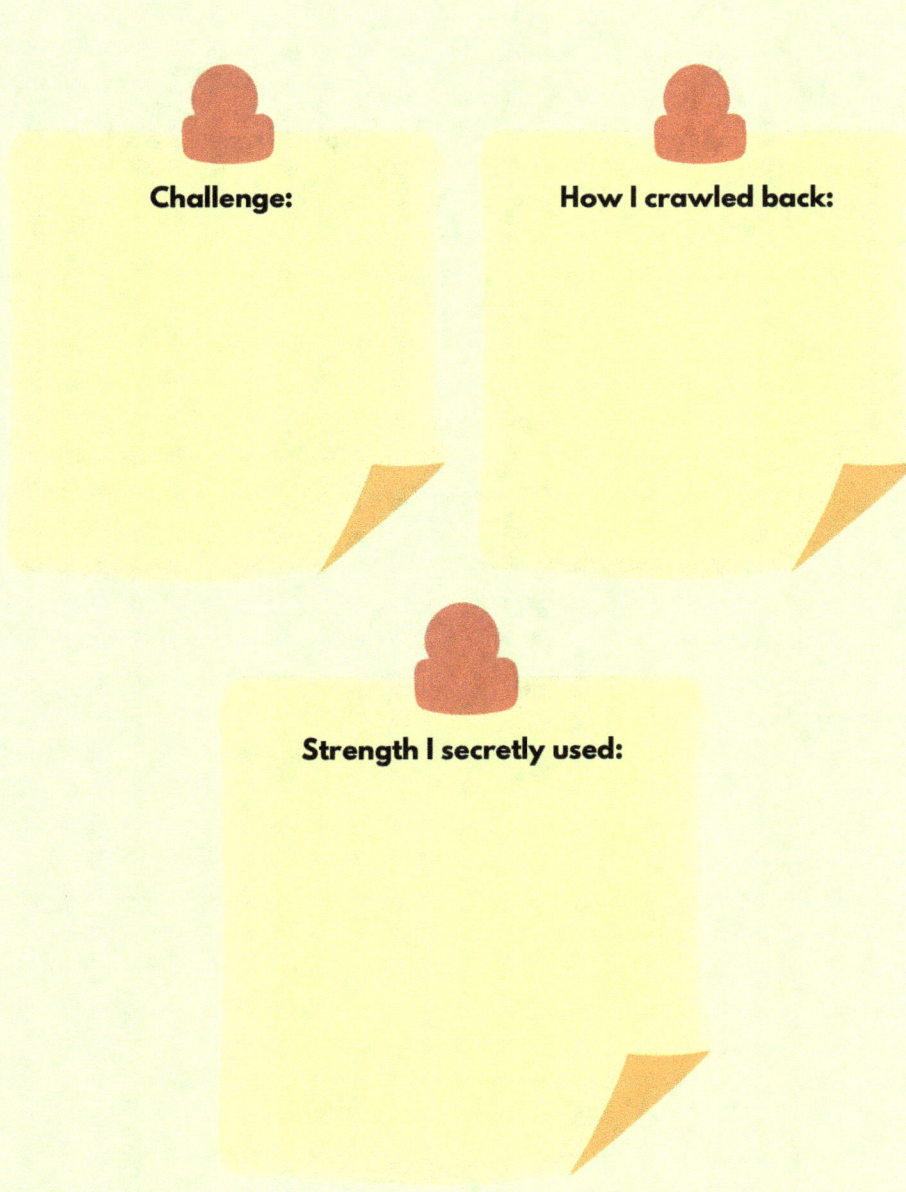

Challenge:

How I crawled back:

Strength I secretly used:

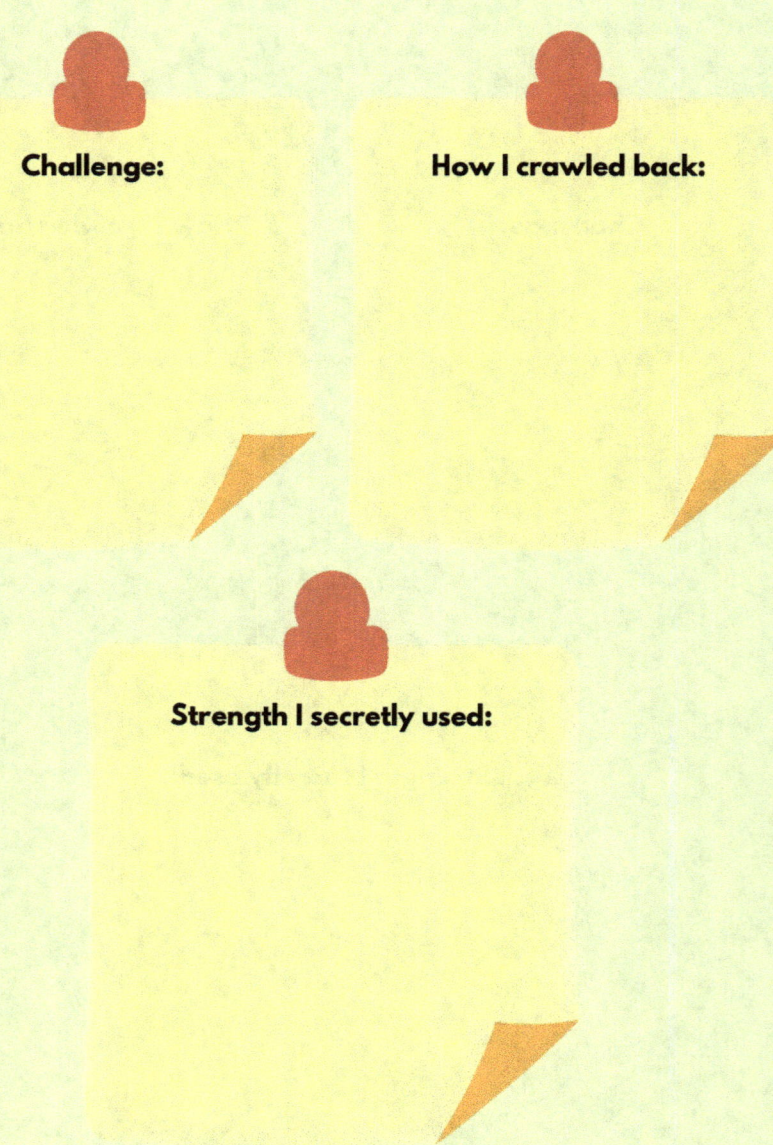

Challenge:

How I crawled back:

Strength I secretly used:

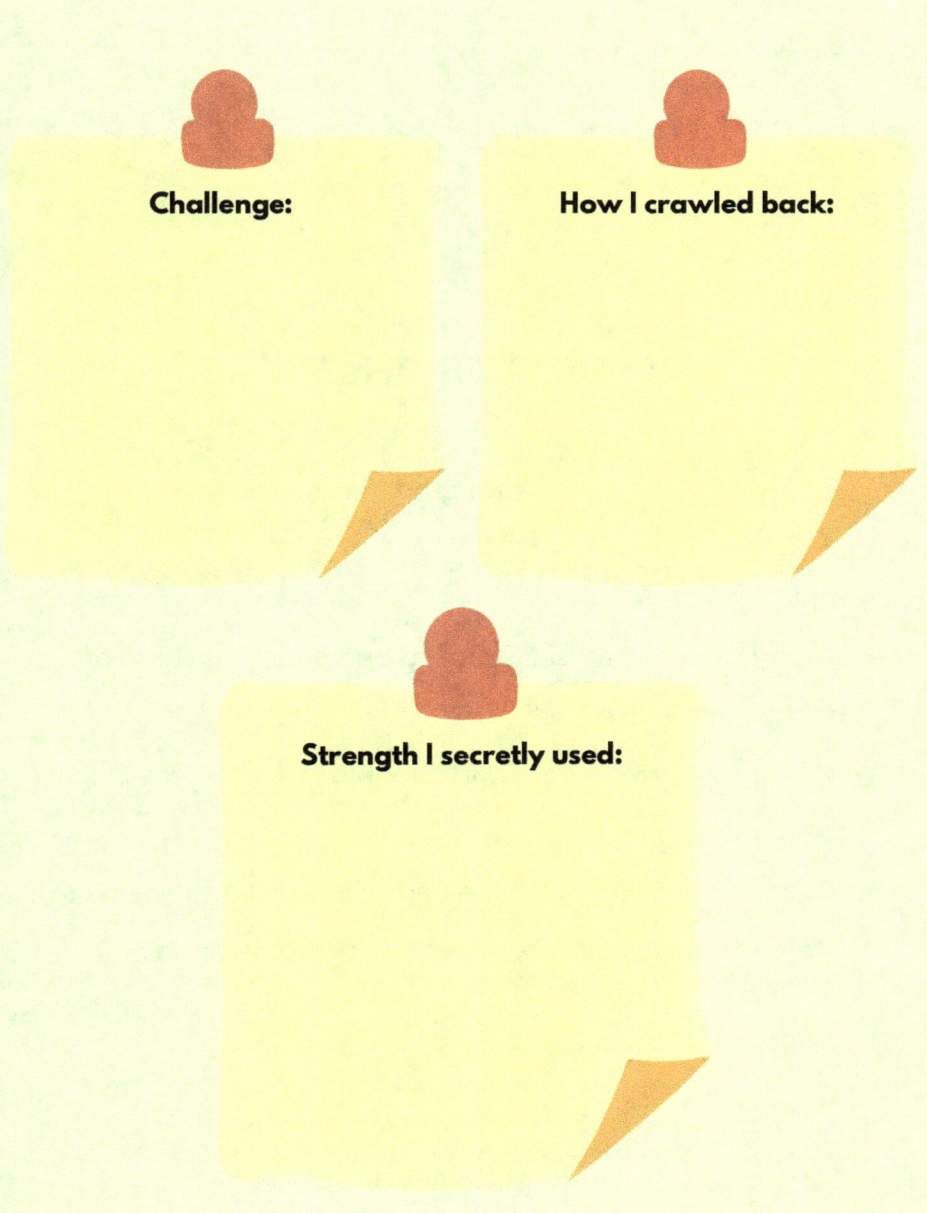

Challenge:

How I crawled back:

Strength I secretly used:

MY INNER STRENGTH

This reflection invites us to notice small signs of inner strength.

Example:

- **Today I:** noticed myself spiraling and paused instead of being harsh with myself
- **This shows I am**: aware and capable of slowing my inner reactions
- **This tells me that:** even when emotions feel overwhelming, I can respond with care rather than adding more pain

TODAY I:

THIS SHOWS I AM:

THIS TELLS ME THAT:

TODAY I:

THIS SHOWS I AM:

THIS TELLS ME THAT:

CHAPTER 11

WHAT HOLDS US IN THE STORM

Don't confuse this with self-worth. The life value spoken of here is the thing that genuinely makes you happy and deeply passionate. It is also a personal compass that helps you know where to go when you feel lost.

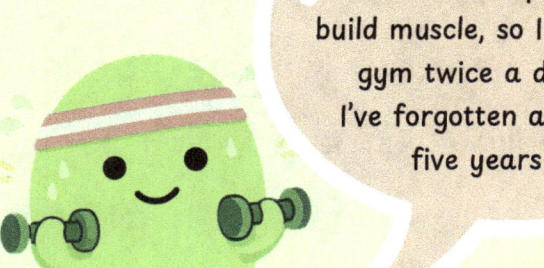

I remember that there was a time when I deeply wanted to build muscle, so I went to the gym twice a day. But... I've forgotten about it for five years now.

So from now on, I'll pursue it, even on the days when I feel sad. And one day, I'll have muscles to show off to my dog.

When stress lasts too long, we often begin to lose both feeling and motivation for life. I once lived with that sense of emptiness from the age of seventeen, an age that should have been full of youthful energy, and yet I eventually lost interest in almost everything.

This chapter offers a simple reflection:
Find again a life value that all those painful stories have taken from you, even if you no longer feel much passion because you are so tired. Or discover a new life value, even if you do not feel much emotion for it yet, and slowly allow a new feeling to grow around it.

Do not assume that a life value has to be something grand or intense. It can be as simple as gardening, learning an instrument, rescuing animals, or even just self-love.

When we reconnect with a life value we once forgot, or discover a new one, we may begin to feel less lost and less adrift in those unanswered questions about our life and the way we see ourselves. Unlike a goal, which ends once it is achieved, a life value is more like a direction we keep moving toward each day and carry with us wherever we go. It can continue to guide us through changing emotions and shifting moods. Even on difficult days, we can continue following our life values so we remember where we want to go and how we want to live.

It may be that when we feel moved to contribute to something greater than our own pain, we are finding something steady to hold onto in our life. I do not mean that we should rely on life values alone in order to keep going, but we can think of them as one of the quiet compasses that help us feel a little less directionless. Remember to do what truly brings us happiness from deep within, not what is driven by someone else's approval or expectations. When we find a life value, we may begin to realize this:

Today I may not feel entirely okay with my emotions, but I still know what matters to me.

To begin reconnecting with your life values, think back to a moment in the past when you felt most alive and most like yourself. It may have been creativity, learning, freedom, self-love, devotion, or something entirely different. Then circle the three values that feel most true to you.

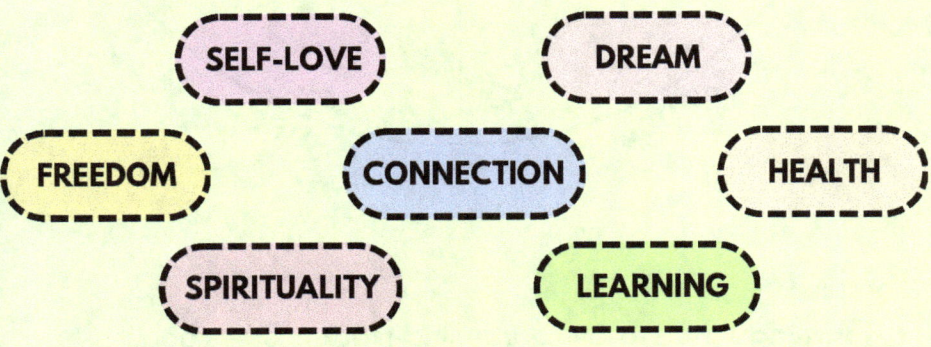

SELF-LOVE   DREAM

FREEDOM   CONNECTION   HEALTH

SPIRITUALITY   LEARNING

**Choose 3 values that feel most "you" and
fill in your actions from the past:**

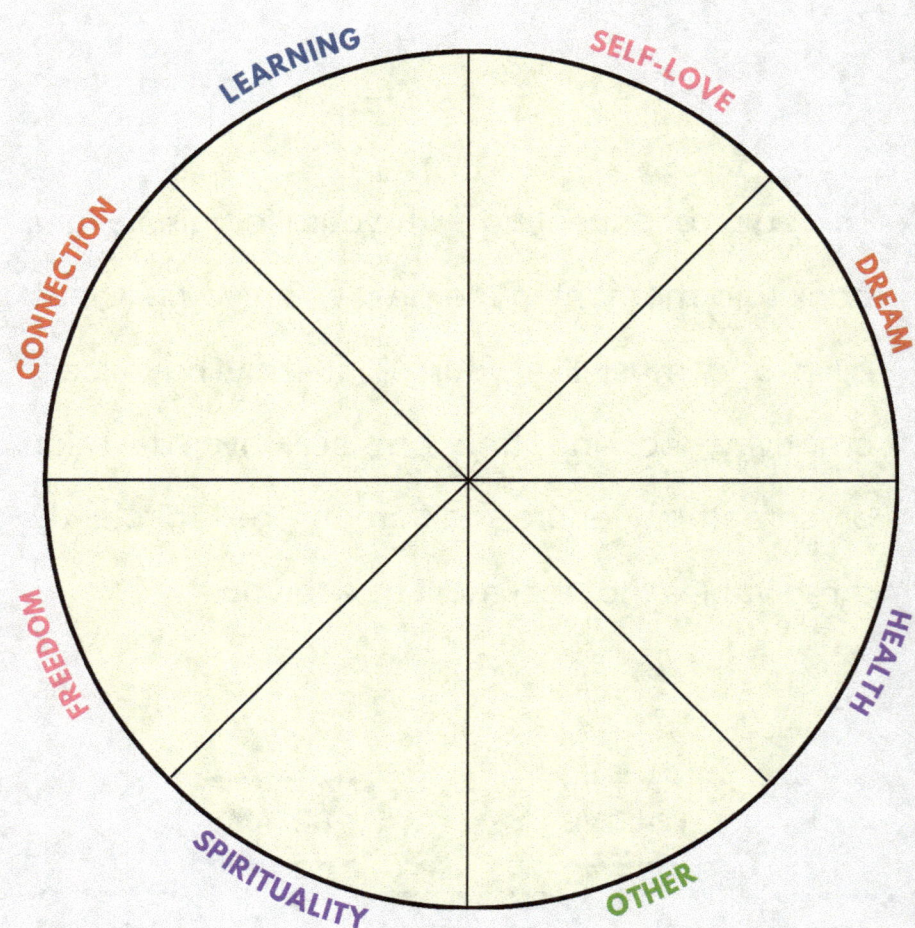

Example:
- **Learning**: I used to love gardening. I took courses about growing plants and vegetables, and I once had a small lively garden of my own that I could watch and tend to every day.
- **Dream**: I once organized a small animal rescue project, and I felt deeply excited and inspired by it.
- **Self-Love**: I used to care deeply about my skin. I spent time taking care of it every day.

Now, instead of asking: "How do I get out of this feeling?"

Begin to ask:

"Even while I'm going through this painful feeling, how can I live today as fully as possible with all that I have, rather than focusing on what I lack?"

This question may open a different inner state, where pain is not the only center of attention.

"Why bother?"

"This matters, no matter how I feel."

The storm whispers:

Values shout back:

Example:
- **Value:** Self-love
- **What blocks this value:** "I feel too tired and it will not make a difference."
- **How I let this value win:** Spend five calm minutes on a gentle skincare routine to refresh and keep skin more refreshed

VALUE:

WHAT BLOCKS THIS VALUE:

HOW I LET THIS VALUE WIN:

VALUE:

WHAT BLOCKS THIS VALUE:

HOW I LET THIS VALUE WIN:

VALUE:

WHAT BLOCKS THIS VALUE:

HOW I LET THIS VALUE WIN:

LIFE MINI-PLAN

Choose 1–2 values and one action each:

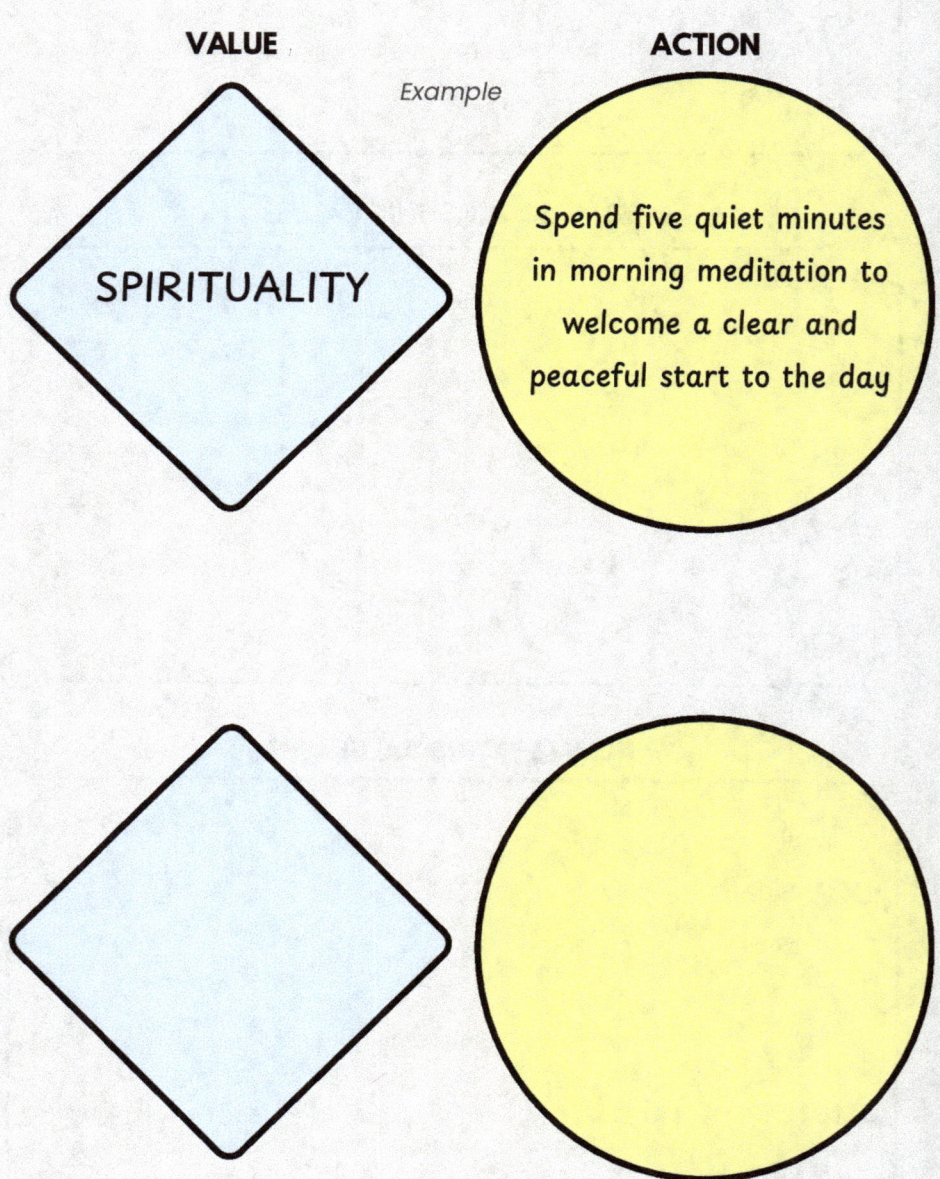

VALUE

Example

ACTION

SPIRITUALITY

Spend five quiet minutes in morning meditation to welcome a clear and peaceful start to the day

VALUE   **ACTION**

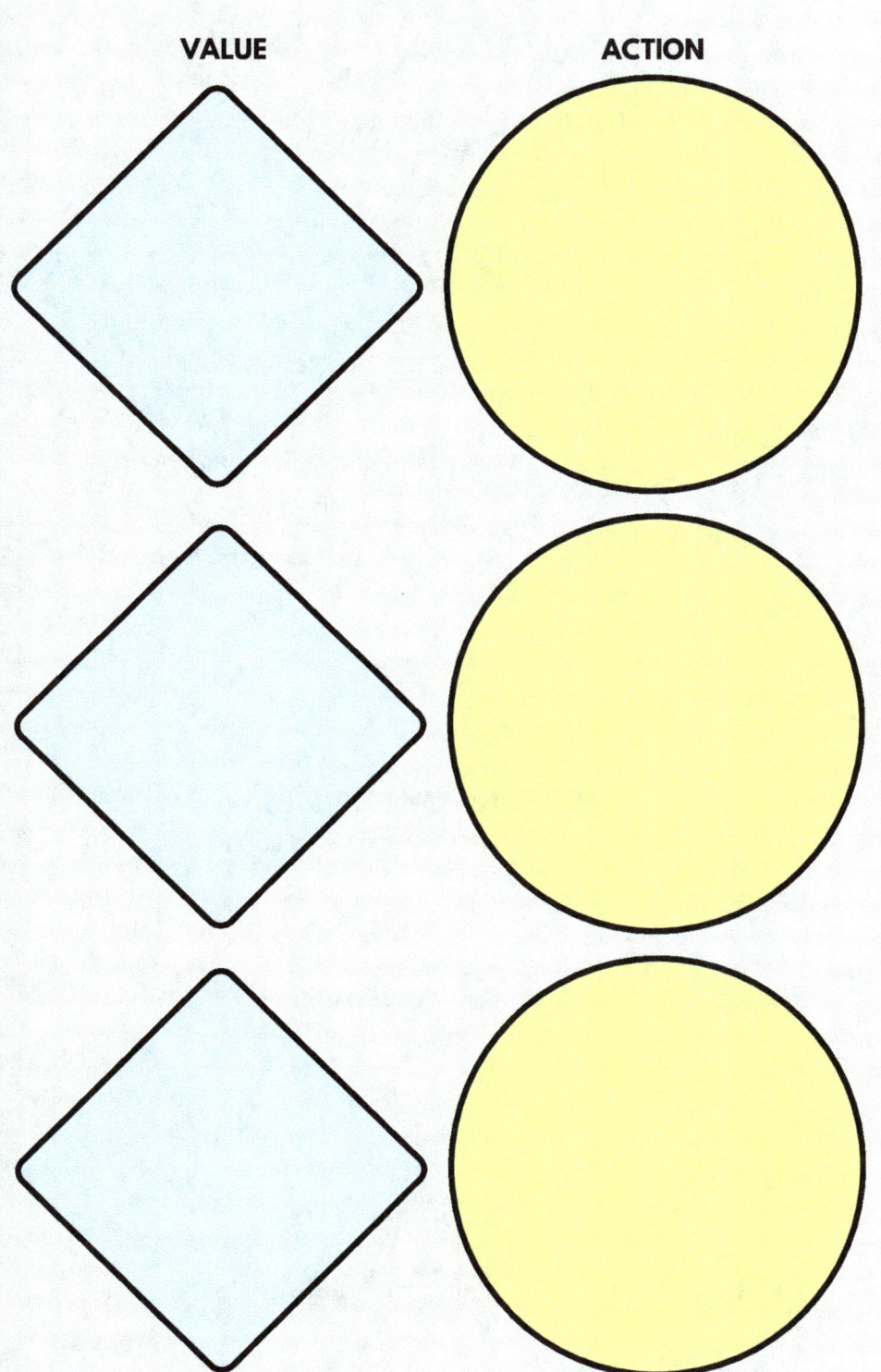

CHAPTER 12

PUT WORRIES IN A LOCKED BOX

Solvable worries:
Real life problems with a clear path toward action.
(Example: "I have a bill due tomorrow.")

Unsolvable worries:
Endless "what if" loops that never seem to reach an answer.
(Example: "What if this feeling never ends?")

SORTING MY WORRIES

Write 2 worries from this week, and sort them:

Worry 1:

....
....
....
....

Solvable or Not?

....

Worry 2:

....
....
....
....

Solvable or Not?

....

Worry:

....

....

....

....

Solvable or Not?

....

Worry:

....

....

....

....

Solvable or Not?

....

Worry:

....

....

....

....

Solvable or Not?

....

Worry:

....

....

....

....

Solvable or Not?

....

ACTION FOR SOLVABLE WORRIES

If a worry can be solved, thinking about it over and over usually only keeps the hamster wheel spinning.

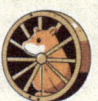

The way forward:
TAKE JUST ONE STEP
No matter how small it is, it is like lifting the hamster out of the wheel.

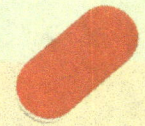

5-STEP PROBLEM-SOLVING

1. Define the **problem** clearly.

2. List possible **solutions**
(silly ones count too).

3. Choose **one realistic option**.

4. **Try** it.

5. **Review** how it went.

SOLVABLE WORRIES

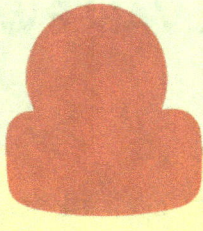

Solvable worry:

....

....

Solutions I can think of:

....

....

....

Solution I will try first:

....

....

When I will try it:

....

....

Result after:

....

....

UNSOLVABLE WORRIES

Putting worries in a locked box, which means placing them outside the center of our attention in a space that may feel quieter, without denying that they are there. So where is that place? We can imagine putting our worries in a cupboard or box and locking it up, especially during moments when we cannot solve everything right away, and then tomorrow, or at another time when we have enough energy to think about it, we will open that box. This image may give us a way to organize them more neatly, set them aside for a moment, and choose for ourselves when and how we want to open that shelf again. This can make the worry feel a little less immediate, as a reminder that it does not have to take up all the space in our mind right now.

**Write down worries and imagine placing them
on a shelf until tomorrow (add "worry time" if you want).**

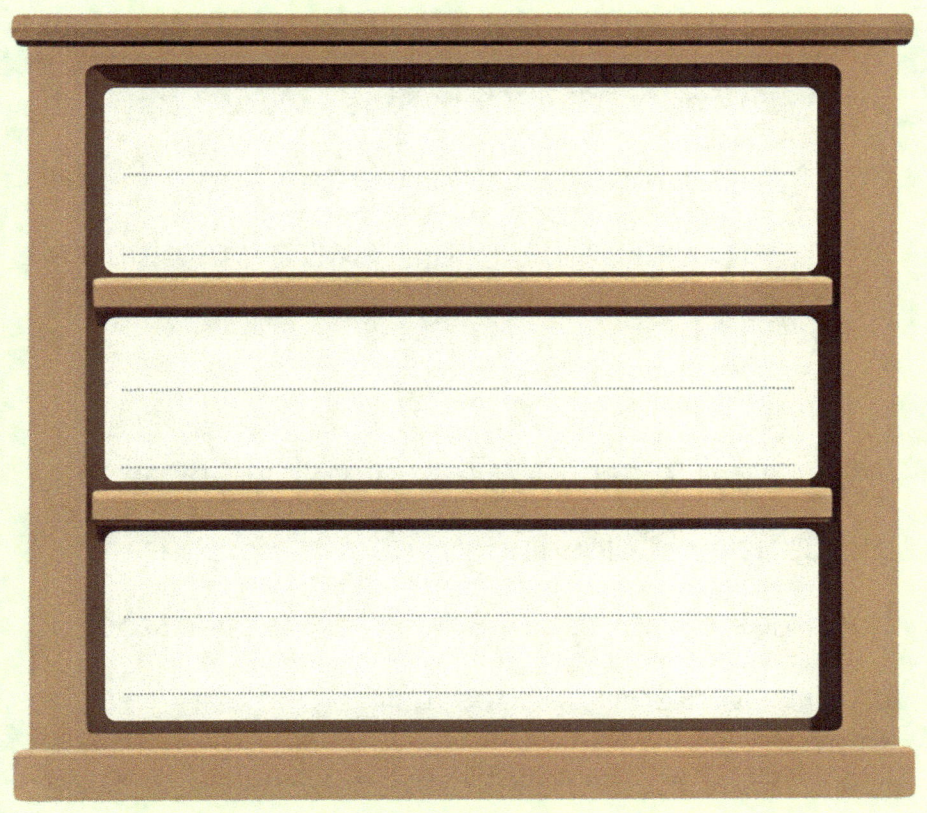

CHAPTER 13

SMALL RITUALS FOR RETURNING TO PEACE

It is hard to tell a person not to think about the past anymore. For someone who has lived through too many storms, the memory of those storms may still echo in their soul, even after time has passed.

When we accidentally stain a wall, we often think about using a cleaning product to scrub it until it becomes clean again. But have we ever stopped to ask whether, besides using a cleaner, there might be another way to make it beautiful again? For example, painting over it with the same color, or drawing a new image over the stain?

There are times when the inner storm becomes so intense that we think peace must be somewhere far away, and that peace can only exist when the storm is "over." One thought appears, then another thought answers it. The noises in the mind keep speaking back and forth until our inner world is filled only with heaviness. And because we want to find stillness, we often try to push away and silence those noises. But perhaps, sometimes, stillness is already beneath the storm, even while the wind is still blowing above it. The question is whether we can pause long enough to see it and feel it.

When we stop chasing our thoughts, when we stop forcing ourselves to feel peaceful, that may be when we begin to feel something that seems still.

What if stillness is not the absence of the inner storm?

This moment is where we are present. We are not drifting into the past. We are not letting ourselves live inside the story of the past.

Have we ever stopped for a moment to ask ourselves whether we have truly returned to the present, or whether we are still allowing ourselves to be swept away into some part of the past? Have we ever wondered whether, if we paused our thoughts about the past and paused our worries about the future, and instead focused only on the present, on listening to the breath of the present moment, we might find a little peace?

Sometimes we are living in the present, but the "fuel" we use to live in the present is still some distant past that has already passed. We keep feeding on it every day and sinking into it, until it quietly nourishes our soul in the present.

When we realize that we are feeding on memories of the past in order to exist in the present, we begin to give ourselves the choice of another direction. It does not mean forcing ourselves to forget the past immediately, or forcing ourselves to become peaceful in a single day. It is more like a reminder practiced again and again until it gradually becomes a habit. That is why creating a small ritual to follow may help us remember what to do, instead of becoming lost in the storm.

Example

If I notice:

A negative thought keeps repeating inside me.

I will remind myself:

This is a belief I learned. It may not reflect the full truth.

My first step will be:

Pause, then respond to the thought with a more balanced one.

If I notice:

I will remind myself:

My first step will be:

If I notice:

I will remind myself:

My first step will be:

MY PLAN CONTRACT

- Every day, I will spend some time reflecting on my inner world so I can understand it more clearly.

- Every week, I will spend a little time taking care of myself, whether to feel more refreshed, or simply to learn how to keep a sense of peace in each breath.

- Every month, I will write down the small achievements I made during the past month, as a way to praise myself for still moving forward, even slowly.

MY PLAN CONTRACT

Each day, I will:

_____

_____

_____

_____

Each week, I will:

_____

_____

_____

_____

Each month, I will:

_____

_____

_____

_____

CHAPTER 14

YOUR PROJECT

When we begin a personal project, no matter how small, it can sometimes offer a source of emotional support, so that hardship no longer takes up all the space in the mind.

I once heard a story about an older woman who sold street food from a cart that stayed open until 2 a.m. in freezing weather. One night, a customer asked her how she could keep working until 2 a.m. in such bitter cold. She answered with a sentence I still remember: For her children, a mother can go through so much hardship and still feel happy. Staying awake until 1 or 2 in the morning does not matter.

Even though each person's pain may be different, and each person's endurance may be different too, that story may help you understand that when we find a reason greater than our pain, our emotions may feel a little less overwhelming than before. Like the woman in that story, she may have felt lonely or quietly hurt at times, and may sometimes have felt unhappy because she could not sleep while the rest of the world was asleep. But even so, she still felt happy.

Beginning a project, or in a less heavy way, simply a small plan, does not erase pain, and it does not mean it will suddenly heal you. Still, it can open up a different emotional current, so that pain no longer takes up all the space in your mind. Instead of asking only, "How do I survive today?" you may begin to sense a future you want to stay connected to. Even on mornings when you wake up with an invisible stone pressing against your chest, your energy drained and your motivation low, knowing that something is still waiting for you ahead can sometimes help you feel a little steadier.

Begin by thinking of something that makes you feel happy or interested, something not tied to anyone else's expectations or standards, as long as it feels positive to you. Or you can return to one of the life values you discovered in earlier weeks and begin shaping it into a small project, whether it relates to a dream, a career path, or simply your inner growth. Then write down why it matters to you. If you feel discouraged and think you cannot do it, do not panic too quickly. Remember that by now you have learned many skills, and you are no longer the version of yourself that had so few choices before. Do not lose confidence just because the echo of past pain is still there.

DEFINE MY PROJECT

Write down one project you want to focus on this week:

Example:

- *Project: Begin planning a meaningful charity project*
- *Why: Because creating something that helps others gives my life purpose and brings lasting inspiration.*

MY PROJECT AND WHY

MY FIRST STEP

Write down the very first small step you will take toward your project this week:

PART 1 – DEFINE THE FIRST STEP

First step:

PART 2 – SET THE TIME

When and where:

PART 3 – PREPARE YOUR MIND

Possible block:

Supportive reminder:

CHAPTER 15

REFLECTION

MY TOP 3 MOMENTS OF GROWTH

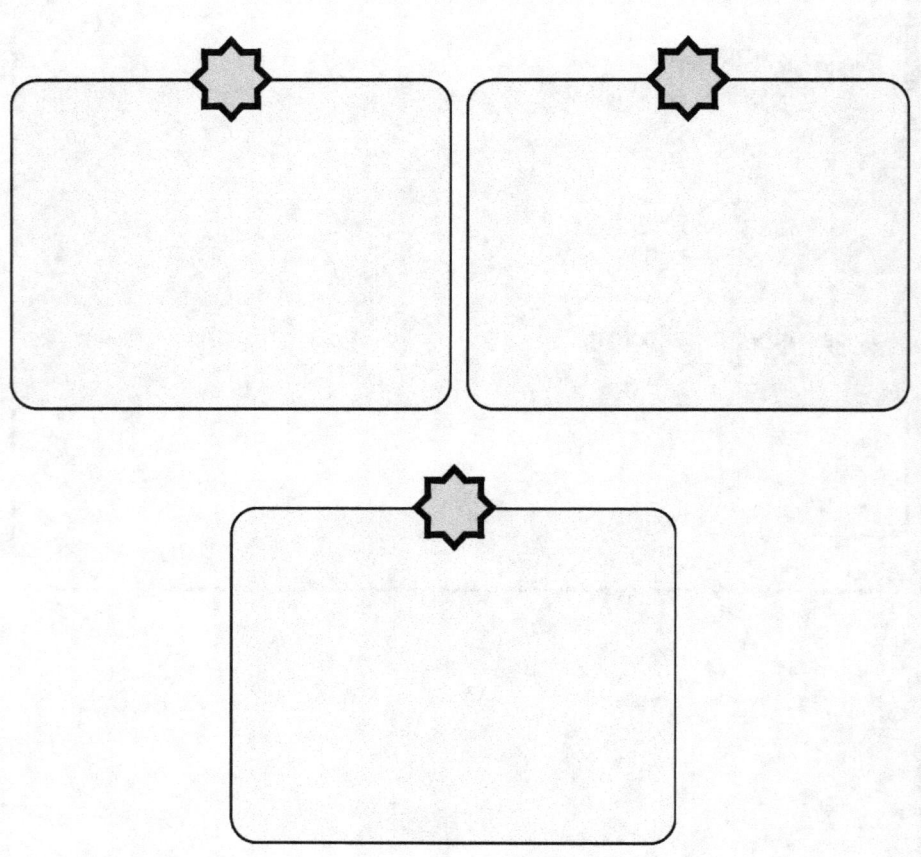

LETTER TO MY FUTURE SELF

LETTER TO MY FUTURE SELF

LETTER TO MY FUTURE SELF

The storm may visit, but it is not the whole sky. It is only one part of the picture.